YOUR HEALTH IS IN
YOUR MOUTH

INNOVATOR PRAMOD STEPHEN

Because of the dynamic nature of the Internet, any web addresses or links contained in
this book may have changed since publication and may no longer be valid. The views
expressed in this work are solely those of the author and do not necessarily reflect the
views of the publisher, and the publisher hereby disclaims any responsibility for them.

The information, ideas, and suggestions in this book are not intended as a substitute
for professional medical advice. Before following any suggestions contained in this
book, you should consult your personal physician. Neither the author nor the publisher
shall be liable or responsible for any loss or damage allegedly arising as a consequence
of your use or application of any information or suggestions in this book.

Any people depicted in stock imagery provided by Getty Images are models,
and such images are being used for illustrative purposes only.
Certain stock imagery © Getty Images.

Scripture quotations are taken from The Holy Bible, New International
Version®, NIV® Copyright © 1973, 1978, 1984, 2011 by Biblica,
Inc.® Used by permission. All rights reserved worldwide.

Lulu Publishing Services rev. date: 10/09/2020

I thank God who has given me Blessing, Knowledge, Wisdom, Talent and strength to write this book for the welfare of the world.

I thank my Father Rev. Stephen Pope & Mother Mrs. V. Stephen Pope who educated me more than their capacity. I am what I am now because of them.

This book was dedicated to mankind in 27th Sodh Yatra on 28th May 2011, Kishan Bhawan, Silli, Randhi, Jharkhand by the hand of respected professor Anil Gupta, I.I.M. Ahmadabad, President.

Siristi Foundation, Ahmadabad (Gujarat.)

PREFACE

BY THE GRACE OF GOD and help of friends and family, I was able to finish this book in 30 years of hard labor's and reading Human Physiology Animal Physiology and Aquatic Physiology. I experienced that God has given different kinds of digestive system to every creature.

I have searched the cause of diabetes and metabolic disorder, reason why it is occurring and the use of only substitutes in this disorder.

Nowadays, this problem is epidemic because it is not only occurring to those who are 40 years old and above but we can also find these disorders in children. For diabetes we use herbal medicine, allopathic medicine, physical lab our, yoga stem cell exercise, and control in food and also other type of system but till date we failed to cure it and people are getting unfortunate death. According to world health organization diabetes is a clinical syndrome characterized mainly by polyuria, polydipsia and polyphagia due to absolute deficiency of insulin or diminished biologic effectiveness of it or both. After a long search I found that diabetes is accruing due to lack of secretions of, cysteine and bile salt in the blood and reduced secretion of bile salt by gall bladder or not prepared by liver by obstruction dehydrate, fasting malaria, typhoid, Kala Ajar and any other reactions that causes diabetes. This definition I sent to World Health Organization in 2006 but they did not send me any comment.

After continued study I change the definition. I worked on new definition of diabetes and people got benefits and they asked bile juice medicine but due to lack of research and law I did not give them. I am also thankful to the Principal of Patna Medical College & Hospital. When I went to him for bile juice script he sent me to Dr. Rajiv Ranjan Prasad of Prof. Human Physiology. He read all my script and appreciated me. Again I went to him to show him new definitions of diabetes then he encouraged me and told me that I will get a noble prize for this definition alone.

I gave my script in the program of Janta ka Darbar mien Mukhya Mantri through district administration. My script went to civil surgeon (District Chief Medical Officer) He read all the script and he appreciated the script He told me that my innovation is quite right but he can't do anything. He gave me letter for Drug Controller office address.

I send all my innovations to National Innovation Foundation. I am very thankful to Prof. Anil Gupta Prof. Ahmadabad and chairperson of N.I.F. I sent my innovation regarding bile juice substance to World Health Organization they advise me to send script in systematic protocol. I am asset less person to fulfill all their protocol. Till now I cannot fill their protocol. Because in the protocol, there are too many questions and tests. I live in very small place and all test laboratory is very far away from my place and it is costly also.

I tried to prove my method in various ways in local standard but was not fully successful. In my mind, there are a lot of things to prove but I cannot do it due to lack of time and money.

I am thankful to my friends who help me. From ancient times the problem of diseases increased and many organizations, doctors re-researching giving many kind of advice like medicine, Health Educations, Yoga, diet chart, physiotherapy etc. but now new disease are coming up and same disease is incurable like diabetes, leucopoenia, asthma, aids and many types of cancer etc. To control this disease all national government and the World Health Organization are spending lots of money but people are still dying. From the last 30 years, I am searching of remedies for diabetes and other metabolic disorders but seeing all medicine substitutes and path and its work. I found that by this kind of medicine substitutes and herbs can only control it but all kind of remedies fail to cure it. I have written many articles and published in many International Medical Journals then

I experimented my method in many patients and found fruitful result and after that, I think to write a book for the mankind.

As we know that our world is going very fast. If we will take example of internet from 2G we can now reach 5 or up to 6 G. If our net is not working and very slow then we get disturb and we feel uneasy. Till now research is going on to make all things fast. We are always in hurry positions and we have no time for our self. It is a big problem for the world and every human because our health is responsible for our every kind of happiness. If our health is disturb then our mind is also disturb and we lose our mind, money, time and work. If one family member is disturb then all family members get worried as well.

We must give time for our-self and maintain a healthy living process. So I start writing a book and it is my first book. I hope that my book is beneficial for all people around the world.

SUBJECT MATTER OF THIS BOOK

1

HISTORY OF TREATMENT

FROM THE PAST OUR INNOVATORS innovated many things and by their innovations our life become comfortable and joyful. By their knowledge, labor and innovative mind we reach the moon. Till now people are doing innovations but we have not reached the perfect knowledge especially in the field of medicine. Our knowledge is not perfect and science does not cure certain diseases.

According to history in 5000 B.C. Mahatma Dhanwantri introduces Aruveda(Herbal). He was the first innovator and introducer of medicine. After that in Aryavarta (our country India) done many research work, Charka, Susrut Vega Bhatt done more work in 800 BC. Mahatma Hunnyman written in his book organ and that, which time people, can operate one hair in 8 parts. This kind of operations, stitching, healing of wounds healing of blood was the highest technology we can see in Mahabharata, people got wounds and all blood was passed away from their body but the next morning all were ready to battle.

In Arvada the main cause of diseases is Bat, Pit (Bile) and cough in this way our body will disturb and the disease will occur. My one invention is by bile juice we can increase hemoglobin rapidly within 8 hours, 2 to 5 grams without any toxic effect. My innovation gets to its peak by Arvada Allopathic. He described that balance diet, clean air and rest is the secret of healthy man. He described that man has self-cure process by nature.

Homeopathy introduces by Mahatma Samuel Fadrik Hunnyman in 1787 to 1789. He described that natural change, character, living standard in the causes of diseases. His treatment is based on the fixed principal of similar. Mahatma Shushlar introduces the Bio-chemic Medicine and he emphasized that in our blood, due to deficiency of salt diseases occur. He described 12 kinds of salts in the blood. But he not described any things regarding bile salt. According to me bile salt is the very important salt for our digestive system and metabolic process.

Instead of it in other country man innovated and develop many kind of Medical Systems. Now many kind of medical system are present in world like Naturopathy, Iso path, Antipathy, Zyso path, Bio-chemic path, Fruit path, Vitamin path, Home path, Homeo path, Physio-science path, Acupressure path, Acupuncture path Spiritual path, Rake path and two by me Chewing path & Bile path.

2

ANCIENT AGE & PRESENT AGE

FROM ANCIENT AGE ALL CREATURE want to live longer and no one want to die. Death is a biggest pain. God created all creatures to die and He fixed death for every creature. I have been searching for the age of human beings in many books and asked many people to know the age of the people in ancient times but till now no anybody could tell me and prove me by any book that in ancient ages people lived for that much age. Only in Bible I got that, all days of Methuselah were nine hundred sixty and nine years and he died. Genesis 5.27 and all days of Noah were nine hundred and fifty years and he died. And Shem livened after he begat Arphaxad Five hundred years, and begat sons and daughters genesis 11.11 and Abraham was one hundred years old when his son was born unto him, genesis 21.5. Altogether Abraham lived a hundred and seventy five years genesis 25.7 Moses was a hundred twenty years old when he died, yet his eyes were not weak nor his strength gone. Deuteronomy,34.17. By above passage, we can see that the age of people become less & less. They were very strong high & healthy. If we will see old arms as seen in Museum we cannot use it properly due to heavy weight because we are not as strong as them. Now our age limit is "Between" 60 to 130.

3

ANCIENT FOOD AND PRESENT FOOD

IN ANCIENT AGE AS WE see in book, people were eating esculent tubes root, fruits and vegetables. After some time they began hunting and only after civilization they began to cook new items and have it. If we would see 50 years back then we find that, that time only plump grains was present like Kodo, China, Marua (Ragi) plumpy paddy. That time there was no new machine for paddy, wheat and pulse, that time people were using stone, pit and stone to clean it or grained it and after some time people prepare wooden parts from that time to this time matter is same but all machine is very fast that time people are using wood and stone by hand or leg its speed 5o times per minute but now a days by machine one thousand per minute and some machine required more than one thousand speed minute. Which reduce the vitamin and minerals from the grain now people like thin flour and thin rice thick grains we are not able to eat for example we can take paddy we will clear clean paddy husk, by hand or Okla. We can found that in side rice is red color now people removing that red color portion by machine called sailor and all good things (bran) they supply for animals and we are eating white rice only. Some kind we are doing with maze and wheat also.

God made some fruit and green vegetable to remove the skin and some fruit and green vegetable we can eat and cooked without removing skin. But because of modern fashion we are removing fruits and vegetable for both. Otherwise, we are taking the juice only. All fibers and valuable things are being thrown away by doing this process.

4

THE IMPACT OF FLORA & FAUNA, AQUATIC AND AMPHIBIOUS IN HUMAN LIFE

DISTURBING OUR DIGESTIVE SYSTEM AND most of people are suffering from constipation. Due to constipation we give invitation to many diseases. Today we prefer liquid food, tasty food, junk food, fast food etc.

In ancient time all fruits, vegetable, grains and esculent rood pulses grow in nature without any pasteurizing and fertilizer. Previous time, the fertility of soil was more but now we can see that the fertility rate or PH of soil become less. Borax, Sulphur, Iodine, Zink and phosphorous this micro substance become less in soil. We can see this kind of deficiency in the fields. Many lands grow very good plants but there is no grain in the plants. In our area Bihar and many places of India this kind of complain is increasing. Before some years we are getting fruits by mango tree every year but now days we are getting mangos alternate years. By this way we can see that all fruits, vegetables, grain, pulses and roots less vitamins and land also get have deficiency of micro substance and for the plant protection we spray toxic medicine to all fruits, grains, roots and plant it's become sweet poisonous.

At present time, agriculture is the main source of human's food. We can see that what kind of seed we are sowing. If we sowing sugarcane land is same but the taste of sugarcane is sweet. If we will sow chili seed on same land the plant grow chili plant. I think that everyone know the test of chili.

It is hot test. We are receiving oxygen by tree and plants in completely different manner, day time it gives oxygen and in night it gives carbon dioxide. After this chemical change air get balanced air of oxygen, carbon dioxide, Helium, Nitrogen and hydrogen. I experimented below a tree and I found that the smell of tree is completely different. For example I went to Neem (the margosa tree) the smell of Neem tree (Azadirachta Indica) is bitter, once I sow Basmati paddy in my field that time the whole field is filled with Basmati smell. We can see that all plants increase the balance of air and along with that they increase our immune system. It's also increases and decrease bacteria, virus in the air.

Just like this flora & fauna and aquatic creature and amphibious creature they belongs to different types and the smell of snake, frog, fish, turtles, cow, buffalo, camel, goat, deer, lion, dog, tiger, bear, cat is different. I found that when fox cries kho-kho at night it produces light (sparking) when lion roars it can be heard about 8 mile away. we can understand that every creature have other kinds of food, sound, smell and it produce oxygen, carbon dioxide, methane and other gases they are all important too.

5

NATURE, DISEASE & TREATMENT

FOR EXAMPLE ALL HERBIVORES PRODUCE more methane gases. It is 2 times dangerous then carbon dioxide but we are producing tetanus, smallpox vaccine from herbivores and many medicine are being prepared from herbivores organism, for example Insulin. When all creature are eating food then food not digested in same types it goes to metabolic process same kind all types of chemical changes take place in air, water, soil, all living creature its requires more research.

Keep in mind that in the nature, (shiristi) knowledge and chemical innovations came to solve the problems of illness. There is closed relationship between diseases & treatment. We can see that, if we will keep water for some days or week the insect developed itself. If we want to observe nature than we must see in the month of February in India, that time if weather is cloudy, then all area of the mustered plant flower plant will be full of Lahi (Aphid) insect. If weather is clean, than this kind of insects will not come. How much this kind of insect develops and they come. We don't know where they come from and where they develop. We spray poison to kill it to protect our crops. When we do not wash our mouth and other part of body then disease comes by itself as mouth disease or skin disease stomach disease etc. when we don't have food at right time then disturbance of stomach comes itself. If we don't take food at right time then bile juice starts to come out and then bile juice start to digest in the duodenum cells and by this process other parts gets affected. When plants don't get water that time they become dry just like when we not eat food that time we face under sickness. We can see the sign of deficiency in the field when potash, lime, Zinc, Boron, Sulphur borax, and phosphorus is not in proper position, then plant gets different colures and plant gets very easily effected. Same kind of sign & symptoms develop in our skin eyes and other part of the body and our immunity power becomes less and infections affect our body easily. God has given all types of medicine in nature.

6

LOGIC OF HUMAN PHYSICAL ENGINE AND MECHANICAL ENGINE

WE ARE UNABLE TO IDENTIFY all medicine. We use different System (path) to control or cures the disease. But we are searching for many diseases. We can see that nature give us disease and quire itself for example we are seeing that when east wind comes we feel pain in our body and by west wind we get relief. Some kind of disease is like influenza, eye disease also today we are doing work against the nature for example we are not walking by foot, not doing exercise, not awaking in morning time. When we work in night time and not sleep at time this is also against nature. Otherwise we are wasting time in talk or watching T.V. of Film etc. other side today in big cities there is lot of pollutions like Air, Sound, Water, Light, Soils, Radiations, Flies, Mosquito chemical pesticide etc. by this things we are fighting with nature by this we are getting sweet poison and slowly its develop serious health problems. Once we see that nature cure the disease itself. For this reason we must live in clean environment clam and pleasant environment must maintain our social order than our immunity power become strong and disease will not come easily.

Take care of nature and its controls the diseases.

From the start of life, human wanted to know things. All human wanted to see new things and learn. In childhood, we can see this habit the most. We observe that when we give any kind of playing items to the children, they play for some time after that they will open the playing things and after that they want to keep the things in accurate place. Many children have this kind of habit. By this habit many children give another shape of the playing things, likewise we see that from the beginning many kind of Machine discovery done by people. Today many kinds of machine and instruments get modernized and many old innovations become finished and many destroyed. For example Sudarshan Chakra, Agni Ban, Uren Khattola, (flying plane) mammy of the Egypt (mammy kept in Miser pyramid) many present in pyramids. It is thousand years old. If we would take example of mummy, now a days there is no chemical or process to keep dead body for thousands years. We can only keep the dead body up to 48 hrs by present chemicals.

Today, new innovations is continued going on as stone arms to stone flours mills, before we can do very little work by water now a days we use Hydro Electric and by hydroelectric we can use in home, big & small factory. By the power of air we are producing electric and using for ground water and other work also.

By solar energy before we are using water heating, pickles, cloths drying meat drying etc., but now a days we are using for solar cooker, solar charger, solar calculator, solar light, solar motor etc. Today steam engine is out of dated, that place taken by crude oil engine, kerosene oil engine, petrol engine & diesel engine. Before we are using wood Cowden for cooking purpose in the stove but now a days we are using Cowden gas. I am using this gas since 16 years.

We see that Petrol, Diesel, Kerosene oil engine process and metal we use is different. Innovators spend time, mind and power to create new machines. There is lot of power in machine man cannot work as machine one. Diesels, Petrol, Electric engine can do faster than human, for example one Rail Engine can run 200 km/per hours in the load of thousand people. That much work 1000 people cannot do. If we take only diesels, engine, this engine is without carburetor. In engine every part is more important and every part have other work as chamber, block, head, crank, connecting rod, bearing, gajan pin, locks, liner, piston, rings, tipit, bush, inlet valve, outlet valve, nut bolt filter Vassar, air cleaner, silencer, governor, fuel pump, head, pipe, high pressure pipe, nozzle, exact valve inlet valve, nut, bolt, oil seal, weight, springs, fuel tank, gas kit, fry wheel Mobil.

If we will collect these things and keep one place we cannot say that it's an engine. If it is not adjust by good mechanic, then it is only a shape of machine. If only one nut is left or not proper tied then machine will not start and if it will get started then it will break the other part. If lubricating oil (Mobil) is not present the machine will not start and if get started the all parts get spoil soon. Timing is not correct then part of the machine will break and in beginning machine will not start, if started then it will give more smoke and not take load, the expenditure of oil will be more and it will not run properly some time fast and sometime slow, just like the spray of nozzle it is not correct and it is less than machine in the start it will be double and if it is more than machine runs fasts and it will break head valve and expenditure of the fuels will be increase. If fuel pump not adjust properly and above process will be continue. Then engine will not work properly. Today people will more concentrate on (motor car) engine factory, home, cloth, cream, powder, massage and unnatural things but we are not giving more important to natural things. We want to eat testy food and any way fills our stomach not chewing properly.

We must take care of our own physical engine (body).

7

THE IMPACT OF CULTURE CHANGED IN HUMAN LIFE

AS WE KNOW THAT EVERY part of world has different types of culture present. Culture affects our individuality, social impact, behaviors, festival and natural activities. Culture depends upon soil, water, atmosphere, rain, and seasons and naturally germinates plants, fruits, vegetable, grains, birds, animals, aquatic creatures, rivers, wells, hills, rock and speaking systems (Language).

For examples in Hindu religion people believe that the creation of earth done by "Berma, this believe depend upon our oldest book "Shamved. In Muslim earth was created by "Allah" they also think that God sent Koran from the sky.

Bible also says that the world created by God and by his word power all things created. The Lord God form the man from the dust of the ground and breathed into his nostrils the breath of life and the man become the living being. Genesis 2.7 Till now, we are searching the origin of earth and all creatures. But we fail the get its answer. In our syllabus we include different theory of evolution without any scientific proof as Lamarck (1744-1829) Charles Darwin (1809-1882) Hugo Deversi (1840-1935) and other person theory also. Now we reach on the Moon and preparing to go to Mars. In medical field we studying genes, the chromosomes, DNA test, stem cells we already Know that we cannot mix two other types of genes chromosomes examples, Goat and Horse, Snake and Crocodiles. We know that if we cross the horse and ass the ass give us mule. But mule have no sperm for other generation same kind of experiments done by scientist they cross lion and panther they got new variety of animal. It was big and very strong but they cannot develop their next generation because the development of reproductive systems is not available in the both sex than how we can believe the theory of evolution and why all world people include their education syllabus. It is wrong concept the local culture system. By reading the evolution theory most of the people become atheist.

By cloning system we producing animals but chromosomes is same as previous animals. We are able to produce plants by leave; branch and other part of the plant, just like test tube baby but all the plant have same character as the previous plant. We can mix two kind of plant and produce new plant but both plant character we can see in new plant, till now we have no any technology to make frog by rat sperm, cell or any part of rat. Then why we include the theory of evaluation in our syllabus and destroying our culture.

According the Are build Garrod 1901 search more than 200 traits transfer in next generation but till now not any human given birth to any types of monkey. I never saw in my life any monkey given birth in human or any animals given any other types of animal than how we can believe the theory of evaluation. In other examples we can take from our country South and North India both of places in puza, devotion and any other program people use the cow ghee If cow ghee is not available then buffalo ghee if both is not available than in south people used coconut oil and north people use mustered oil it is depends upon availability of things. In north people are using mustered oil. I went south India their food I don't like because of smell, in Bihar people cannot drink coconut tare. South people drink coconut tare. If Bihar people drinks coconut tare then disease will developed. Bihar people using very less tamarind and south Indian people much tamarind and they give rasam as a respect previous time in

Bihar people using only vegetable and sweets in marriage party. But in Bengal fish must be in marriage party. It is a custom but now days all the customs and culture has become a mixed culture.

In Bihar, people believe that water of Ganga is holy and people used in pooja, (devotion) and in last time of life they give Ganga Water. It is our culture just like Kaveri River, Neel River Shiloh kund (sink) etc.

Today we see that for employment people goes country to another country then they learn their language, cloths wearing styles and culture those are not fit for our culture. For examples we will take Punjab State Bihar people will speak their language styles and they think that it is very good for us but is wrong for our people because in our area we are using "Aap" as a respected word and "tum" for little children, but in Punjab people are using "tusi" word for all as in English we are using "You" for all if the use the word "Tum" (you) for respected people then the feel very bad and for some time people will get shocked.

In India there are very cold and very hot places, we wear clothes according seasons but in fashion. During hot season many people are using tight cloths and after some month people will get skin disease due to heat and sweat.

8

FOOD, DISEASES AND TREATMENT

WHEN SNAKES TRAPS THE FROG then it became very lazy and becomes heavy. It cannot run fast, thus people and other creature kill it very easily. God has given it very good digestive system. Snakes can digest whatever they swallow. But human digestive system is not like snakes or other animals. When human eat more than they can eat they will experience indigestion and most of the people vomit it or out it by mouth. Or will be suffering from vomiting + diarrhea. We eat food to get energy and when we eat too much, it could upset our stomach. Then we lose our energy and to correct the stomach, we have to pay for medicine. By this process we lost our energy, money, time and mental peace also. When we go to marriage functions or any other function then we do not get food on time and in function we eat more and we give invitation to the disease by this way we see that we get toxicity.

We don't take same kind of food always we must change our food because by this way we will get vitamins, minerals etc. we must include pulses, rice, wheat, vegetables, flowers, roots, leave, tuber roots and dry fruits in our daily food. By this process the minerals and vitamins required by our body will be fulfilled.

If we have required food, than we will be healthy. If we have more food, than we will become sick.

.

9

PHYSIOLOGY OF HUMAN, DIGESTIVE SYSTEMS

GOD HAS GIVEN DIFFERENT DIGESTIVE systems to every creature. Some has only mouth not teeth, some have more teeth & some have beak. Some animals eat once in a week, some eat for one month, some eat for six months for examples Bear and crocodiles eat for six months. Some animals digest their food by bile juice; some animals digest their food by bile juice and bacteria. For examples carnivores digest their food by bile juice and herbivores digest their food by bile juice and bacteria. We can see in human we found gallbladder but in horse they do not have gallbladder only liver is present, we do not found liver in earth worm this way we found that every creature have different digestive systems. For every creature some organs are responsible and every part of body related to digestive systems.

ORGANS, RESPONSIBLE FOR DIGESTION

1. Lips
2. Teeth
3. Tongue
4. Muscles of Cheek
5. Gums
6. Gland of Mouth
7. Gland of neck.
8. Stomach and it muscles.
9. Liver
10. Bile and gallbladder
11. Pancreases
12. Duodenum
13. Small intestine
14. Large intestine
15. Anus and other

Other organs which affects our digestive systems:-

When we are worried or very happy, we do not easily get hungry. When our blood pressure becomes low or high, we get hungry. When we have any trouble urinating, we lost the feeling of hunger. If blood leucocytes, Eosinophil's, and E.S.R. increased that time we lost our hunger. If we have lung infection and less oxygen in our blood we can see effects in our digestive systems and restlessness also. When glucose level increases in blood, we feel more hungry. This way we can see that above organ affects indirectly in our digestive systems and this effects gives us bad effect in our digestive systems and metabolism.

CLEANNESS AND DISEASE

The meaning of cleanness

1. Pure Hearted
2. Cleanness of environments

3. Cleanness of home area.
4. Cleanness of body.
5. Cleanness of Stomach.
6. Cleanness of cloths and external part of the body.
7. Cleanness of internal part of body.

1. **Pure Hearted:** We have to keep our heart clean and pure, because if our heart is not pure our brain does not work properly. If we have fear in our mind and our face does not look cheerful, our every organ of the body is physically affected. When we are afraid, our digestive system and every gland of the body is physically affected. For example if we have done some mistakes and we feel guilty, our eyes becomes down. So my advice is keep our self away from sinful nature like sexual immorality, impurity, debauchery, hatred, discard, jealousy, fits of rage, selfishness, ambition, dismiss ones, factions, angry, darkness, orgies and other evil works. But fill yourself with love, joy, peace, patience, kindness, goodness, faithfulness, gentleness, and self-controlled. Then when you look cheerful, by nature your immunity power will be increased and you will be healthy.

2. **Cleanness of environments:** We must keep our environment neat & clean. If our environment is not clean then we cannot keep our self-healthy. We need air to be alive and when we breathe polluted air, viruses, bacteria and dust goes to our lungs. For example when we go to a mining area, we will feel suffocated. A lot of people are hospitalized for TB in industrial area because of the types of dust that are present in the air like, carbon dust, stone dust, glass dust, mica dust, coal dust, lime dust, etc.

3. **Cleanness of Home area:** The cleanness of home means the cleanness of channels. Boots makes house environment beautiful because in boots there are many kind of insects, flies, mosquito and other types of fungi developed. We must clean water cooler. Outside of the house we should plant some flowers & trees. By these things our heart become happy and we can get oxygen,

shadow, fruits, flowers etc. The home decoration must be done and everything should be kept in proper place and that gives us good look, when we enter in home that time we feel happiness.

4. **Cleanness of Body:** Naturally some salts and chemicals came out from our body daily by sweat and dust collect in our body. If we will not take bath for one day then we feel uneasy and sometime we feel pain. For example in our genital organ, there will be like lime substance collected if we do not clean it regularly then it produces smell and if we do not clean it for long time then it produce some pimples and afterwards it become disease. Same kind of substance collected in our mouth and tongue also when we wash our mouth and clean the tongue that time we see it clearly. In nails there is some particles also collected we must keep our nails clean and cut it regularly.

5. **Cleanness of Stomach:** There are several steps and processes that could aid digestion. We should drink plenty of water. Fiber and vegetables must always be present in our daily food diet and we should take time to chew our food. Because of this, our food are being digested very easily and all the necessary vitamins and minerals are being absorbed by our intestine and our body gets the full energy from the food we eat. There are a lot of people who have done this and they told me that it was easy for them to defecate and their stool are very clear I will say that it is very good process to keep our stomach clean.

6. **Cleanness of Cloths and external part of body:** We must wear clean and dry cloths. We can see many people mostly in villages where they clean clothes in river, tank and water pump and take bath and after bathing they wear half dry cloths. I found out that after some time they get skin diseases and because of the moisture they will get backache and other pain also. We should wear cloths according to the seasons for examples according to Indian rules advocate most wear black coat for their identification in summer seasons. I found that in summer season they are sweating and they

feel uneasy so my advice is we must wear clothes according to seasons and we must chose colors which gives happiness and peace.

7. **Cleanness of internal part of body:** It very difficult process to keep our internal part of body and organ clean. We can experience this when we drink less water that time our urine color become yellowish because our body and internal organs need water and they re-absorption of water from our urinal bladder takes place and urine become less and yellowish color. Same kind of process works in energy also. When we eat regular food and we eat more calories we cannot expand that time our calories collected in the body in the form of fat. If we will not take food for long time that time our body utilizes stored fats as energy. So my advice is we must take balanced diet as required

For the body and drink more water to keep our internal parts clean. We should live where there is fresh air and exercise regularly because from our body carbon dioxide comes out through our breath and we required oxygen and because of less oxygen our body feels laziness and our brain and other parts do not work properly. So my advice is for purify our blood and got oxygenated blood we must exercise in morning and evening time because in morning time the environment is very calm and all dust and particles was present in air they become clean. So, my advice is for healthy life we must maintain above mentioned process.

10

FOOD AND SOUL

THERE IS AN OLD PHASE that says "As you eat grain so does your thought" means according to your food, our nature, soul, heart and work will be created. I always serve cows and drink milk. I experienced that the smell when we bath cow is of same kind which comes out in my hair and body that means whatever we eat, the substance reaches our tissues that has an impact in our body smell, nature, thought and work. We see that carnivores are more hunter, murderer and filled with anger than herbivores. We observe the same kind of nature's we can see in humans which directly impact in our heart we found in our life that without any reasons we feel anger, un-satisfaction, and evilness. This way according to our thought, heart effects in our digestive systems. For examples when we are angrier than our body hair will be stand we feel dryness of mouth, blood pressure become high, voice is also changed and after some time there is no voice in our neck and after a long time we talked in loud voice then we get pain in our neck. It will continue for more than one week and we take medicine and do gargle it will shows only external type of abnormality. But we cannot see that our slavery gland and tissue gets effected or not our internal gland how much effected.

After some time we find that our stool becomes dry or we get diarrhea. By this fact we can see clearly that food impacts our health and affects our digestive system.

11

DISEASE AND DIGESTIVE SYSTEMS

THERE ARE MANY KIND OF disease in digestive system but I have divided it into only two parts.

1. Temporary digestive problems.
2. Chronic digestive problems.

1. **Temporary digestive problems:** Temporary digestive problems comes for few hours as burning sensation in stomach, acidity, gasses, boils in mouths diarrhea, Vomiting etc.

2. **Chronic Digestive problems:** The Chronic Digestive problem comes for a long time. A swelling in intestine, chronic pain, piles, peptic ulcer, intestinal tuberculosis, Liver Cancer, Pancreatic Cancer, Tongue, Cancer etc. Temporary digestive problem comes for few hours or for little time. The reason is human eat more food, eating late, sometime people eat old food, empty stomach, worms in intestine, eating food without chewing, useless food extra.

Chronic digestive problems- Many people keep worms in their stomach because they do not feel any problems. Like hookworm, tape worm, round worm, thread worm, ameba, bacillus and other types of worms. By this there are many kinds of disease occurs in long time like gastric, pain, dysentery, peptic ulcer, erosion of intestine, intestinal tuberculosis, skin disease and effects of worms disturb our metabolic process and due to disorder of metabolic process many people gets white patches because of hookworms sucks the blood and when they reach near the skin they use dope, dope + melanin gives color to our skin and except this worms gives many kind of skin disease like eczema intestinal problem, liver problem, gallbladder problem, pancreatic problem and other problem also.

If we take only piles, there are various cause that lead to piles which ranges from edge starting during bowel moment, constipation, dysentery, lifestyle, low fiber diet obesity, coughing, or liver diseases some other conditions that can leads to development of pile include hypertension, premenstrual syndrome all these situation leads for pile. Junk food, less chewing of food materials, High blood pressure, causes pile. But my opinion is that only due to constipation piles occur. We must change our habits of eating food & water more chewing then our bowel comes out very fresh and we will be free from piles and other stomach disease also.

12

MOUTH

MOUTH OF EVERY CREATURE IS more sensitive under mouth, lips, tongue, Teeth, muscle of cheek, gums etc., our every part have function to excrete and absorb. for example, when we bath in the river that time we feel thrust and urine, because our skin absorb water in our internal part and then excreted by kidney and collect in urinary bladder we don't know that what is our hair absorb but in plants we do not know that thorn is absorb water by air. So according to my lips also absorb and excretes. For example when we smoke cigarette we feel bitterness in our lips and we feel that place heaviness and whole mouth, lips, teeth, tong, gums becomes bitter for few hours. It's my personal experience including three people who smoked. I told them that smoke shouldn't be taken inside the lungs etc. They experience that the carbon was being collected in the lips, teeth and whole mouth become bitter for two to three hours. So my advice is to wash mouth after eating anything mostly after eating sweets in night time. We must wash mouth before sleeping.

13

TEETH

IT IS MORE IMPORTANT PART of body. Because by teeth we are chewing any kind of food without teeth our voice is not properly come out. Our teeth control our tongue and give tongue to move in proper place. Otherwise our tongue does not work properly. We can see in old aged people that some time we don't understand the voice. Teeth control anything to go inside and outside the mouth. By teeth our face looks beautiful. Teeth work as a protector. Teeth control both jaws. By our long bone marrow produce red blood cells. By this we cannot understand our teeth secreting any substance because our teeth are very sensitive place, it must prepare some substance who gives the strength to digest food, and we must read it. We found that in young stage if teeth broken down by some accident or any reason then our digestive system become weak. We can see and experience it when any people fighting and playing if we want to expand our full strength then we must keep our teeth tight. Teeth keep in teeth tightly it will give us full strength. If there are no teeth in our mouth then our strength becomes less. Many times we our teeth as a protector instrument by biting. This way we can see that teeth impact our digestive power, physical power and protection power. It is my opinion that teeth secrets phosphorus and mixed in saliva and keep metabolic process correct. Because when we use artificial tooth then then we feel some disturbance in our mouth and we cannot chew food nicely as we chew by natural teeth. We see many people save their teeth for hundred years and till death his or her teeth become same as young stage because they maintain their life style. So, my advice is to all people brush your teeth after eating

Any food mostly after eating sweet and sour things not brush to much because the upper part of teeth enamel gets lost and teeth feel severing and we feel upset when eating & drinking anything.

14

PROCESS OF BOWELS

BOWELS MEAN CLEANNESS OF STOMACH. If our stomach is not clean that time we feel many kind of disturbance in body. Many people stop their stool and they do not go in time by this reason stool become dry and it develop constipation and sometime stomach pain and severe pain. If this process continue for some months, its, develops gas, piles, headache and metabolic disorder. In many families we can see that they have big houses but they have no toilets and many places we can see attached toilets and bathrooms, both are not fit for good health. In the village who has no toilets they go outside in open place for toilets, their man can go any time for bowels for women only two times morning and evening because their nature is feeling shy. If women gets bowels day time she stop their bowels and by this process they will get headache, backache, indigestion, dryness of mouth, stomach pain, gas and many kind of problems. They go to the doctor, doctor gives medicine, they get relief for some time that problem is as it was. The reason is they control their bowels, in many places we can see room attached toilets many people not go for walk they spend their all-time in home then due to less exercise our body metabolic process get disturb and people gets disease. We must de worm our self after six months and morning and evening must go for toilet. Today there is no time for toilet when pressure comes than only we go to For bowels. We can see in old age our (Sadhu), Saints what time they go for toilet nobody can see. They get up early in the morning and do all cleanness and they prepare themselves for work. But today we are looking TV up to 11 to 12 PM and get after 8 AM no time for morning walk. Now we can see that people waiting for bowels (pressure). Somebody drink tea, coffee, using cigarette, tobacco it is become our nature. Without Tea, Coffee, Cigarette etc. people cannot go toilet. It is like a disease. Previous time people go for bowels in the field and when they go that time they keep scarping instruments (Khurpi) and they dig a pit and after bowel they filled it up. By this way they save the environment and make soil fertile. My Mother and Father teach me in my childhood my all brothers and sisters done this process. Today I did not see this kind of process. Because, we have no facility to do these process, in town? But we can use it in villages. Now we can see that near the village or small town roads is full with stools and our mind get disturbed by smell and by motor and any speedy vehicle it will go to some people cloths and our leg, shoes, sleeper gets dirty. It is a big problem for every Village and small town and some big cities also. Now we can see the fashion of attached latrine and bathroom in the bedroom for cleaning it we are using insect sides and many kind of purifier to remove the bad smell. By this way we are using sweet poison and our nature become disturbed and we are not taking fresh air in morning time there are many kind of toilet sheet but we are using mostly two types of sheet one is that we can sit on it like sitting in field and another is like sitting on chair or stool. Commode is very comfortable but in long term it is harmful because I show many people

15

SYSTEM OF BATH

WE CANNOT SIT AND GO anywhere without chair shape commode go for toilet because in chair type commode our leg is not getting proper exercise in long time we can see that human cannot sit in the toilet he do stool in half bow. By this way we can see all the previous system changed. So my advice is we must change our daily routine and go for bowel morning and evening. *We must keep teeth to teeth in tight position at the time of bowel by this process our teeth become strong and durable as my mother told me.*

From old age to till now the source of water is river, tank, lake and rain. There is no change in natural reservoir only change is taken place in underground water because we are using underground to much by hand pump, tube well, etc. When we go for bath or any animal or birds go for bath then first leg go in the water, by this process we make our body tolerate the water temperature and the leg temperature reach to the head by blood circulation. Till now we enjoy swimming in swimming pool, in river, sea, lake & tank also. But more people are not getting this kind of time and place to enjoy. Only they use tap water, hand pump water and nowadays in every place the fashion of artificial spring is going on. When we open it then water directly comes on our head and our whole body feeling swearing and after few minutes or second the body becomes normal and able to tolerate the normal water temperature. Nowadays it is the big problems for good health and other problem for middle class people they are using artificial tank and tap water in the winter if becomes very cold and summer season times it becomes very hot. To control it we are using water heater and for hot we are using ice or frieze. By this process we experience that some time when we use hot water in heater water, become hotter and when we drop water in our body we feel very uneasy for few minutes or seconds. We feel same kind of experience when we use cold water.

16

PROCESS OF FOOD

IN BIG CITIES PEOPLE CANNOT live without fridge because hot weather. Many people given time for bathing are 4 o'clock to 10 o'clock and much other idea present in the world. In modern age every place we are using bathroom. But in old age and my childhood I am bathing in open air. And till now, I prefer open air bath in Tank, Rivers, springs and other open space. According to my opinion 5 to 7 o'clock morning is the best time for bath because this time whether is clean clam and Sun should be read and by the sunlight our body gets vitamins A + D naturally. And if our body lacking any type of color it will be fill naturally.

In ancient age our forefather and monk had food in very calm and quiet place. Our Rasht pita Mahatma Gandhi also did the same. He made special room for eating that called "chowka" (dining room). That room was made only for eating purpose. Not any other work done in that room. In that time he sat along in that room and had the food and enjoyed it. In these days all over the world the process of eating is changed. Today people are eating with family not in dining room but in drawing room. They listens radio program; they watch TV while taking food. By this process we cannot concentrate our mind on food and enjoy food. Previous people believe in simple food and high thinking but now a day's people like tasty food and spicy food. Simple food and boiled food is out of fashion in every place. We can find only junk food, fast-food and other type of food in Hotels, Restaurant etc., they are more costly but not good for health. Previous people they not eat more spicy they use spices for the treatment like Golmirch(Black pepper), Sauf, (Aniseed)Azwain, (Thymol) Haldi, (Turmeric) Jeera(Cumin-seed) etc. and till now we are using it as a medicine and spices also. Previous people were not eating chili but now day's people using lot of chili. Eating time they drink water many times. By water construction of food digestive enzyme, secreted by our mouth gland and stomach gets disturbed and food not digest properly. If we will eat hot food or more chili that time it is necessary to drink water. Previous people eat the food in sitting position like Sukh Aasan(one type of Yoga) exercise. Sukh Aasan is to sit on the mat or floor and folding both legs but now a day's people need dining table and chair. By this process our folding capacity of knee become less and after long time people cannot sit on floor. It is my advice please sits on the floor while eating and concentrates our mind on food; enjoy the food by more chewing. We must eat food at time because if we not eat food at time then we feel acidity; gastric, peptic ulcer and much other discomfort arise in long time. We can see in marriage time or any other occasion when more people gather in one place then we never get food in time and we feel weakness, trusty, and hungriness and when people get food then they eat food very fast by this process many people get stomach upset, vomiting, diarrhea etc., so it is my advice to people when they arrange any type of party they must arrange all things in time then people can enjoy their food and when people enjoy and eat the food by more chewing then they eat less food.

17

SLEEP

FOR GOOD HEALTH WE NEED good sleep that means not sleeping too much or less we must take good sleep between 6 to 8 hrs. In 24 hrs., In present time we are living in the modern age and in modern age there are lots of industries, hospitals and call centers their people must work day and night and government make rules for a man work 8 hours a day but we can see in govt. and private both places people worked 24 hours continuously. There is no sleeping time. If a person worked continuously 24 hrs. then they get acidity in stomach and his or her metabolic process get disturbed. In the industries and hospitals people work night shift and they got many kind of disorders. If we will go north pole to south pole then we will get trouble because we will get timing changed when north pole get day that time south pole gets night so I found that when south pole people comes in north pole area that time they get one to two month to adjust the sleep because time is day & night totally changed and in north pole people working in north pole place but they work in night that time they also get disturbed because in day time in sunlight they cannot take rest as a night because god made night for sleep and day for work.

And when we not take needed rest in night time then we gets disturbance of stomach. But when we cannot do today the need of people to work 24 hrs. because we cannot stop industry and we cannot close hospitals. It is necessary for good to sleep in right time 9 P. M. and best time for awaking is 5. A. M. It is very old phrase is Early to bed early to raise, Make a man healthy wealthy and wise.

18

DIABETES, THYROID, HEMOPHILIA, CANCER, PILES AND DISTURBANCE OF DIGESTIVE SYSTEM ARE NOT A DISEASE

TILL NOW MEDICAL WORLD DO not accepts that diabetes is a disease because it is not developed by any virus, bacteria, bacillus, worms and germs etc. But we see only clinical syndrome develop and we can find metabolic disorder in diabetes. Some kind of disorders we can find in thyroid, hemophilia, eliminia, mental disorder, blood pressure, cancer, stomach upset, heart attack, insomnia, my Loma, thalassemia, osteoporosis and disease of bone. It is develop due to work against natural law and change in daily routine. When we leave without nature then many kind of syndrome comes out slowly in our body. For example people who lived in big cities are not enjoying nature. There leg never go in to grass. In front of his or her house, only roads is present and they walk on the road, they works in office and they die in the hospitals. Same as chicken, they borne in hatchery they developed in farm they lay egg in farm and they go directly to shouldered house. Not any single farmer left the chicken to enjoy the nature. Same kind a lot of people in big cities not being able to enjoy nature by this way people get same syndrome in long term.

19

THE REASON OF DIABETES AND CURE PROCESS

I HAVE EXPLAINED IN LAST chapter that diabetes is a not disease, only a clinical syndrome and metabolic disorder due to lack of insulin in our body. This enzyme prepare in our pancreases. Pancreatic disease so it is necessary to know the structure, function and enzyme secreted by pancreases. The pancreases is pale yellow gland which is found in reason of the junction between the stomach and duodenum. This has specialized glandular cell that seems to be developed as specialize outgrowth of the gut endoderm and differed histological from the pancreases tissues. These cells an endocrine function, have been known as islet cells of Langerhans. These islets cells were not connected to the duct systems through which the digestive system pancreatic juice flow instead there secretion are freed into the blood circulation. In the pancreases there are three types of cells are present.

1. Alpha cell
2. Beta cell

3. Delta cell.

1. **Alpha cell:** This cell secretes glucagon's this Harmon's converts liver glycogen to glucose.

2. **Beta Cell of B. Cell:** This cell secretes insulin to convert access food glucose in glycogen that is stored in the liver.

Delta Cell of D. Cell—D Cells produces gas tin. It is similar to hormones produced by stomach. It is very small in amount.

As we know the Beta Cell of pancreases secretes insulin. Insulin contains three types of enzymes.

1. **Amylase:** Amylase converts all starch in to maltose.
2. **Trypsin:** Trypsin converts peptone into amino acids.
3. **Lipase:** Lipase converts fat into glycerol and fatty acid.

The function of this enzyme to converts carbohydrate (sugar) into energy and after energy it converts in fat. The impact of carbohydrate (sugar) is less in our body. We are not able to get energy.

If we will see our body upper side than we can find that God have given us two eyes, two nasal cavity, two ears, two hands, two testicle, two legs, and two breasts. In internal part of our body, two lungs, two kidney, pair of internal glands. Even we find two lobes in liver also. If one failure, then one works. God given single part of our body like tongue, esophagus to anus one tube, one spleen, one gallbladder, one pancreas. If we will remove the gall bladder due to infection or hyper cholesterol, the stone is formed. When a person get gall bladder operation the bile juice from liver directly goes to duodenum by hepatic duct that means God gifted something extra to manage the problems, if arises.

If we will see in our mouth and examine the saliva then we find that in our saliva water, Amylase, Lipase, phosphate, Muncin, Mineral salt, liysome, urease, Adolage, Cholestorolage, Iodinase lead mercury, all enzymes are needed for digestion and keep metabolic process accurate. But we don't know importance of saliva. Saliva kills all bacteria, virus and other parts of harmful germs present in food and other drinking materials.

In diabetes chapter it is necessary to know about carbohydrates (sugar). Carbohydrates (sugar) are compound normally characterized by having carbon, hydrogen and oxygen elements in their molecules in which the ratio of the hydrogen and oxygen is the same as the water (2:1). There are exception to this for example, pentose sugar of the nuclei acid, DNA which have formula C6H10O4 there are also a very small number of carbohydrates that contains nitrogen.

The basic units of the carbohydrates molecules are known as monosaccharide and glucose. Carbohydrates are very important wide sprayed biological compound as they are chief source of energy and structural constituent of the protoplasm. They are defined and also structural kitone derivatives of the polyhydroalchohals or in other words the carbohydrates are poly-hydroxyl aldehyde or poly Hydroxyl kitone. They are presented by an empherical formula.

In general carbohydrates are white solid sparingly soluble inorganic liquids but except for certain polysaccharides soluble in water. As we know carbohydrate (sugar) is the main source of energy keep in our body has less carbohydrate (sugar) then we feel weakness and if it is more than body requirements we become faint and if it's become finish then we also finish (dead).

The impact of more carbohydrate (sugar) in our body in above I explain that neither due to lack of insulin nor produced by our pancreases the symptoms of diabetes develop. And lack of insulin the metabolic process of to change carbohydrates (sugar) in energy and fat. If this process not works properly we feel lack of energy in our body and slowly we become weak. Our blood pressure become unstable, Urine trouble, heart problem, atrophy of muscle, eye problem, sex weakness, infertility, ulcer and healing process also disturb. Hormonal disturbance, immunity power, internal gland will get effected and day-by-day we become weak and whole body become ill.

Note: The people are taking any kind of medicine can do this process by taking medicine and after some time they will become less depend on medicine and after full confidence and medical checkup they will leave medicine. They must observe their health regularly.

The following endocrine glands and enzyme are responsible for the diabetes:

Source	Enzyme	Activator
Pancreas	Lipase Amylase Phospholipids	Trypsin
Stomach	Trypsin	Entropeptidase
Mouth Lingual glands. Salivary Glands.	Lingual Lipase. Salivary Amylase	

Besides these enzymes, there are also some enzymes which description is not suitable here.

WHAT IS CHEWING, MASTICATE AND GRINDING

In chapter six logic of human physical engine and mechanical engine we show that if fuel pumps fire inadequate fuels that time nozzle cannot make nice spray. If Spray is not in proper balance according to the liner, piston then engine not run properly, if it is less than engine will not get started and if starts run slowly, if it is more than machine run very fast. Just like God made our hand as a fuel pump, and our mouth is nozzle. We masticate food by hand and mixed with other material and then take inadequate mixed food and masticated food in mouth and grind it by teeth in the form of spray then all food stuff mixed with saliva and it is very easily digest and as we read earlier all needed enzymes for digestion and body requirements mixed in swallowing particles. If we will do this process than our bowel become very easy. The work of any kind of nozzle is to make liquid in the form of gas or spray. We must logically think ourselves that how much we are using our hands and teeth to grind our food and how much we make liquid in our mouth.

HOW WE CAN CHEW THE LIQUIDS

We can see in the petrol engine we are using petrol with mobile oil. This process we are very easily using in scooter and motorcycle. Any person take 5 liters petrol then he must mix 100 ml of mobile oil. By this process the efficiency of petrol become more smooth and durable. It is the experience of Motorcycle Company, motorcycle driver and other experts also. When we drink water, tea, coffee, fruit juice and any other liquid, then we swallowing it directly in this way the saliva not mix in the liquid so my advice is when we take any liquid in mouth then not swallow directly we must keep the liquid in mouth and move the liquid in the mouth or gargle it and enjoy it and then swallow it. By this process all adequate saliva mixed with liquid. There are many benefits of this process as the erosion of esophagus, ulcer of stomach, gas problems, problems of digestive system and its increase the function of internal gland and you will get natural insulin and other enzymes needed for the digestion and metabolic process, your bowel and urine become very easier and you will never get constipation & dry stool. You can examine yourself that how much you can chew food materials & liquid. If you will get constipation or dry stool that means you not chewing properly. If you will get any stomach problem that mean you are not chewing properly or you are not taken food in time or you eaten something else that your stomach cannot digest the material. We know that nature or God given a process to every creature to survive in according to the climate, environment nature we see that every place we found different kind of tree grass plant vegetables and animals birds fishes and insects and we see diseases we find also take place according to climate for example leprosy, diarrhea dysentery is more than cold place. same kind of digestive system we find in herby boras and corny boras both digestive system is different herby boras digest the food by bacteria's and by ruminant process and they gets many kind of vitamins by ruminant process but for Carnivorous digest food by bile juice and very less saliva many creature trap their food and sallow its example frogs and many creatures. human has also different kind of digestive system man has two kind of digestive system (1) saliva (2) by bile juice

Saliva – We know that our saliva contain many type of enzymes and digestive juice vitamins and Using a single saliva sample from a healthy, nonsmoking male subject, the researchers were able to identify 102 proteins, including 35 salivary proteins and 67 common serum proteins. Identifying all of the serum proteins present in saliva could take many more years. With advances in instrumentation, it is predicted that the number of serum proteins identified in saliva will increase significantly, although it will probably never match the number of serum proteins found in blood mainly because serum proteins are only a tiny part of saliva, described as a dilute, watery solution containing electrolytes, minerals, buffers, and proteins. Blood tests are a well-established, proven methodology, and it may take some time before saliva tests can become as reliable as serum tests. In the future, patient and doctors can look forward to more saliva-based tests.[We must masticate food not less than 70 to 80 times in our mouth and we must eat our food for 25 to 30 minutes because in our body some hormones takes 20 to30 minutes to secretes. For example we can take leptin hormones it takes 20 to 30 minutes to secrets this hormones responsible to send a message to our brain that our stomach is filled or we are satisfied with the food. We see that people have no time for food and they finish their food within 5 to 7 minutes and there is no proper saliva mixed in swallowing food and there is no secretion of leptin hormones and no massage come out to our brain then we eat more food. As result many kind of hormones enzymes and vitamins will not function properly and our swallowing food lacking many types of things presents in our saliva. We should not talk at the time of eating because by this process our saliva disturbs and our metabolic process is also disturbed badly. We must chew the food water and any liquid and take meal timely by this method we can cure any kind of metabolic disorders and by this process we can make any kind of food more nutritious because all substance present in our saliva mixed in our foods.

New Definition of Diabetes Given by Me Diabetes is a clinical syndrome and metabolic disorder occurring due to less chewing of food materials and water. According to the All paths of medical world says that diabetes is not a disease then what is the treatment of diabetes? It is metabolic disorder and we can cure it. To correct metabolic process we need to chew our food well as this will eradicate diabetes as well.

20

THE PROBLEM OF THYROID AND CURE PROCESS

IN THE LAST CHAPTER WE show that the problem of diabetes and how we can cure it by natural process. Now we will see regarding the thyroid problem. The problem of thyroid we can divide it in to two parts.

1. Hypothyroid
2. Hyperthyroid

In both circumstances they give bad effects in our every part of internal and external body.

1. Hypothyroid: The sign, symptoms and complications of hypothyroid in human predictable consequences of the physiologic effects of thyroid hormones. The syndrome of adult hypothyroid is generally called myxedema, although the term myxedema is also used to refer specifically to the skin changed in this syndrome. Hypothyroid may be the result of a number of disease of the thyroid gland or it may be secondary to pituitary failure. (Pituitary hypothyroid in completely athyrotic human, the BMR falls) The hair is coarse and sparse, the skin is dry and yellowish (Carotenemia) cold is poorly tolerated, the voice is husky and slow, the basis of the aphorism that myxedema is the one disease that can be diagnosed over the mobile. Mentation is slow and memory is poor and in some patient.

There are severe mental systems (myxedema madness). Children who are hypothyroid from birth are called cretins. They are dwarfed and mentally retarded and have enlarge protruding tongues and pot bellies. Before the use of iodized salt become widespread. The most common cause of cretinism was maternal iodine deficiency. Various congenital abnormality of Thyroid function that cause goiter can also called congenital hypothyroidism with cretinism.

2. Hyper Thyroid (Thyrotoxicosis): Hypothyroid is characterized by weight loss nervousness, hypothalamic, heat intolerance. Increase blood pressure a fine tremor ore of the outstretched fingers, warms soft skin, sweating and basal metabolic rate high. It may be caused by a variety of thyroid disorder including in rare instance benign and malignant tumors. Before highlighting the thyroid disorder we must be aware of the iodine which is stimulate or secret of thyroid hormones. Human mouth (in saliva) there are many kind of enzyme are present as amylase, lipase, phoshotate, lysomacid, adolase, cholestorase, maltose, catalase, urease, protease, iodine, mercury and leads. But in our medical field they only give importance of Amylase and lipase. We must know the importance of all enzymes secreted by mouth are very necessary for the digestion and keep correct our metabolic process and all secreted substance absorb by our intestine. Our internal gland also secrets many kind of hormones our body requires iodine in micro quantities by this hormones

Thyroid gland stimulated to produce thyroid hormones which we can commonly get from vegetables, food and fruits. But in some cases land have no iodine, because of flood and heavy rain all iodine leached out of the soil. That area requires iodine treatment in soil because the deficiency of iodine in soil decreases the yielding process and that area goiter is common. Before 40 years it is more in many places in the world but by the recommendation and help of world health organization (WHO) government solved the problem of goiter. They put iodine in salt. But now a day's new problem arise (Thyroid Problem). This problem is generally in the world. Till now we treat it by thyroid hormones pills. Day by day new problems arise, we are using substitute of metabolic disorders. If we will examine ourselves and iodine deficiency found than it is my advice to treat the soil by iodine instead of iodine salt. Then we can get natural iodine by grains, vegetables & fruits. As I explain above iodine is also secreted by our salivary gland and absorb by intestine it has more important for the function of metabolic process. We must eat food and water more chew as advice in the chapter of diabetes.

Chew your food to protects you from thyroid Disorder

21

CANCER CURE PROCESS

AS WE KNOW THAT ANY person suffering from cancer than we understand that he or she has very less life. Cancer- known as a killer disease in the world. This disease progress differently over a period of time but certain characteristics that include development within any tissue of a malignant growth & erosion divide from abnormality of the host. The abnormal cells grow without any control invades through normal tissue barrier, spread too locally and distinguished within the host and reproduce indefinitely.

In other words we can say that incurable wound; extra growth of tissue and erosion of tissue is cancer.

Why these abnormal tissues developed? Tissue erosion and incurable wound take place.

There are many kind of cancer in the world. Bur we can see how cancer take place in body.

1. We purchase cancer (we invite it)
2. Cancer due to metabolic disorder and hormonal disorder.
3. Genetic Cancer.

1. **We purchase cancer:** We are using cigarette, tobacco, alcohol, opium, heroines and other types of drugs for intoxication. These types of intoxication damage our tissue and impure our blood. When our tissue gets damage, our fibers tissue repair the effected part. This process continue going on. By this reason we gets incurable wounds, hormonal disturbance, metabolic disorder and abnormal growth of tissue in our mouth, lungs, liver, stomach, neck and other part of the body. In last stage it is declared as Cancer.

2. **Cancer due to metabolic disorder and hormonal disorder:** We do not take care of our body as food, types of food, the process of eating, nutrition, exercise, cleanness, process of toilets, process of bath, sleep etc. we fail to maintain natural and social order by this reason there are several disturbance comes in our metabolic process. For examples blood cholesterol, diabetes, thyroid problems, loss of appetite, indigestion, diarrhea, vomiting, dryness of mouth and many kind of problems generated in our body. For deficiency we are using only substitutes. By substitutes we get relief for a certain time. But some deficiency again and again in our body. Our internal organs get affected as liver, heart, lungs, kidney, ovary, testicles, pancreas, spleen, pituitary gland, thyroid gland affected. Sometime tissue collected in our particular part of body. This kind of glands has trouble free sign and symptoms so people are not visit the doctor. When peoples gets pain in gland that time they go to the doctor, that time is too late. Same kind of hormonal disturbance

3. Comes from the childhood to the end of the life. We can see in childhood many children suffering from lymph nodes and in teenage teenager suffering from gynochemestia and after that people suffering from breast cancer. Ovary cancer and protest cancer. This kind of cancer commonly find in people.

4. **Genetic Cancer:** When any patient comes to the doctor they asked two types of history. (1) Disease comes from generation to generation. (2) Disease does not come from generation and not even by mother and father by birth.

(1) **Genetic cancer:** When we asked his history of Heart attack then people says that our forefather also died by same kind of disease. We commonly say that this disease is genetic. But for heart attack protein kinase C is responsible. Till now, we can-not find that when the protein kinase C secreted and how to prepare it. Other factor also gives heart attack as hyper cholesterolemia, erosion of heart muscles, thickness of artery & vain and blood pressure etc. All factors responsible for heart failure and we commonly says that it is genetic disorder or hereditary factor.

(2) Disease does not come from generations and not even in Mother and Father. Till now Albinism known as hereditary. But I saw that it is not hereditary for example: Near my home one family is present named Shankar Ram, wife Bachiya Devi (Changed Name) both have dark color (Normal). They have seven children instead of Seven three have albinism and rest four are normal. One son and one daughter get married. Daughter has five children and all are normal some have one child she is also normal. Then I can says that albinism is not hereditary albinism is disorder of pigments and dope due to metabolic disorder or lack of enzymes in genes. By this deficiency child born colorless his or her body hair, eyes is not normal as mother and father whole body is colorless. If whole body is colorless then they get in this trouble whole life they cannot tolerate heat and cold. Now it is a biggest problem same kind of problem arise in the present world like Thalassemia, My Loma, Leucoprosis many kind of blood disorder in the world. Why this problem arises and developed. Now days, the main reason we are not giving proper health education to the children there are many Health Education Guide. But chewing process is taught, only by me. So my advice is to all children and especially couples that must maintain their good lifestyle, from before conceiving to child birth and thereafter whole life.

22

GENETIC DISORDER

GENETIC DISORDER IS GENETIC MECHANISM transmitted by parents to offspring. It carries the disorder generation after generation. The hereditary units which are transmitted from one generation to next generation are called genes. For the study of genes we have to study nucleic acid and chromatin.

There are two types of nucleic acid. DNA and RNA is the chemical basis of heredity. The study of DNA (Deoxyribose nucleic acid) RNA (Ribose nucleic acid) reproduction, hereditary traits and genetic code is very long process. We must know that when we see any old friend's children then we can understand something by his color, face, habits, walking styles, speaking styles, hairs, body cuts, leg, nail, eyes, skin, lips, nose, forehead, ear and neck. But it is very long process to know about his or her habits, genetic disease and knowing him or her, internally. In previous chapter we show that our living standards like how we eat in ancient age food, present food, natural disease and treatment, cleanness food and disease, food and heart, disorder of digestive system, sleep, process of toilet, process of bath, logic of human physical engine and mechanical engine, the reason of diabetes and cure process, cause of thyroid an cure process, cancer and how we overcome by the disease by natural process. We can ask ourselves that by knowing way or unknown way we are producing new generation in disease less or with disease.

As we know that every living creature need food and water (Moisture) without food and water they cannot survive, God given different digestive system and metabolic process. When any creature keep food in mouth that time the process of digestion begins and all part and gland become active, Mouth to anus and all part of body gets energy. Man is a social animal and all creatures not wash their anus why?

We see all animals and creature look very neat and clean only when they get digestive disorder that time only they look dirty and only that time we found stool in anus and back side. Why because their stomach get upset they get lose motion or constipation. In constipation some stool in anus and lose motion It will spread in tail, legs and body also. Human always using water, toilet paper, leaf etc. Because, our stomach is always gets disturbed. Stomach is the main place of digestive system and stomach affect all our metabolic process. That means if stomach get disturbed then our metabolic process automatically disturbed.

Pedigree analysis show, that habits and character in heritance of traits regular transmission generation to generation and controlled also.

According to Sir Archibald Garrod (1901) suggested that some of metabolic disorder, which were inborn are genetically controlled. He further suggested that such disorders or disease are inherited in accordance with Mendelian laws. The inheritance in human beings follows those same patterns which govern the inheritance in other animals and plants. Over and above, two hundred hereditary trails have been reported to be transmitted from generation to generation in man.

Today all people are more hurry; we want testy and fast food. We do not care for nutrition value of the food. Only we want to fill our stomach and go for work, business and entertainment. Due to work load, ragging by co-workers, fear of boss, teasing other, jealousy, unsocial work, politics, show ourselves big, air pollution, water pollution, hurry to catch bus, train, office. We are always in tension How to earn money. Now traffic jam is also a big problem in all cities, sound pollution, the light of motor vehicle from opposite side, work load more than eight hours, night duties, minerals deficiency, deficiency in grains, fruits, vegetable, drug resistance, drug addicts, pollution of river, tanks, pesticides, synthetic milk and other items prepared by synthetic milk radiation by mobile and other modern equipment's and other luxurious equipment's. Plastic production use of fertilizer except natural manure and green manure all affects our natural cure process and metabolic disorder. Due to lack of time people are using packed food, fast food, pieces food, and food in liquid food, fruit juice and other types of drinks and they are taken in hurry and run for desire work. This kindof our habits, change in our nature and daily routine. As told by someone Habits is second nature. It is very old phrase this kind of habit and nature transfer to offspring by genes. By these habits many mother birth still baby, many mentally retarded, physically handicapped, many children get dead after birth. Many children were born as an Albinism. Many disease and sign and symptom developed after birth till sixty years.

This problem is like an epidemic in the world so I advise to every person in the world that they must eat by my technology to every children, new couples and every person to eat food and water more chewing as explained in diabetes chapter then only we can enjoy our healthy life and then we can give the good health to next generations. By this we can make metabolic disorder free to next generations.

We must turn to nature itself to the observation of the body in health and in care dieses to learn to the truth.

God Bless with all kinds of happiness & health to you and your generations.

23

SUCCESS OF WORK INNOVATIONS DONE BY ME AND ITS SUCCESS

MY FIRST INNOVATION IS LOW cost animals feed by immature paddy:- what is immature paddy? Immature paddy is fly by air or when we keep paddy in water for making saila rice and beaten rice then all immature paddy swim in water it is collect by people and thrown as useless things. It will take long time to become manure and its smell is very bad and when we burn it that time it will give very bad smell just like alkali. Our nose cannot tolerate it. I saw it in huge amount in various places. I saw it from many years and asked people the use of it. But no any single person, farmer, and other person told me to use it. After a long time, I brought it free of cost at my home and grind it in flour mill and then given to my cow as an experiment. My cow eaten very eagerly and then, I given in some more amounts and after some month, I fell that it is useful for all cows. I use it about 10 years for my cows and, I asked for the test in many organizations. But they not told me any appropriate place to me. After a long search and journey; I found a place where my sample was tested and then I got good result by this way my first innovation get fulfill. I sent my innovation to NIF and they select me for Siristi Samman 2007when I got siristi samman then my interest gone very high for new innovations. From that time, I continue thinking for new innovations. By this way, I reach in this positions to learn experience and write for the benefit for the mankind. I am very thankful to NIF because of his efforts and encouragement, I got new vision for innovation's

24

INNOVATION: TREATMENT OF EVERY KIND OF ANEMIA BY BILE JUICE

INTRODUCTION: AT PRESENT ACCORDING TO medical study many chronic disease cannot get cured process. In this present symptomatic treatment without much investigation on the root cause of illness we are using only substitute of the deficiency and only control process going on in the world. But can-not cure. My objective is towards the cure process of chronic disease by bile juice substance.

Our focus is on: deficiency of vitamin *a, d, e, k,* hemoglobin, insulin, disorder of blood and other endocrine gland.

Deficiency of vitamin minerals and enzymes are one of the distrusting conditions in the world people life since long back. Why? When we give the substitute of deficiency we repeat the substitute again and again the deficiency not lead towards the permanent solutions that means there is defective in the absorption or misbalances in the blood, because blood is only processes to neutralize whole tissue of the body and gland.

Why we need this substance: When function of liver is depressed by injury, any disease or by the establishment of ECK's fistula the output of bile salts reduce by 50% These evidences show that synthesis of Bile Salts place probably only in the liver. If a man or animal liver not function properly then the bile salt become less and the absorption of Iron Vitamin A.D.E.K fats do not take place and the Deficiency of above Vitamins disease take place and the cholesterol in the blood become increase and pancreatic function is also affected.

What is anemia: It the red corpuscles loss in the blood due to malnutrition M.C. and Iron is not being absorb by the intestine that is called Anemia. There are many kinds of anemia.

How does the Bile juice work in anemia: If the deficiency of Bile occurs that time the absorption of Iron not take place and the deficiency of Iron Lead to Anemia, and Bile Juice have Bile Salt, bilirubin and Biliverdin. Bilirubin and Biliverdin give direct color' to blood and latter is used in the formation of fresh HB and Increase the Liver function and when Liver function is OK then our Intestine start to absorb Iron substance. We can use it in many' kind of blood related diseases.

Hen: The Gall bladders is about two to three inches long and one inch in diameter & it's filled with Bile juice. It is little thick than goat's weight about seven grams to twelve grams.

Goats: Goat's gall bladder is like egg shape containing about four hundred to seven hundred grams of bile juice and all other creatures have gall bladder according to their body weight and size.

Bile juice is an alkaline viscous yellow to green bitter fluid (ph.) six to ten. In some animals it is secular organ attached to hepatic duct and some birds and animal Attached with liver. During digestion the gall bladder contract and supplies bile juice rapidly to small intestine by the way of common bile duct. The pancreatic secretions makes with the bile since they empty into the common duct shortly before its entry.

SECRETION BILE JUICE

Contraction of gall bladder and relaxation of its sphincter are initiated by Hormonal mechanism. This Harmon cholecystokin It is secreted by the intestine in response to the presence of food mainly meats and fats. This hormone stimulates the gall bladder to undergo rhythmic contraction. These results, in an increase in the rate of flow the bile juice into duodenum. The gall bladder bile juice is more concentrated then the hepatic bile. In the Gall bladder water is observed and mucus is added there for the bile juice concentrated and. becomes viscous fluid.

COMPOSITION OF BILE JUICE

(1) Mucin Or Mucus
(2) Mineral Salt
(3) Bile Salt
(4) Bile Pigment
(5) Cholesterol
(6) Lecithin
(7) Fats & Fatty Acid
(8) Water

(1) **Mucin or Mucous:** Secretions contain mucopolysaccharides as those from of goblet cells of the intestine. The sub maxillary glands and other mucus glandular cells. Mucin also present in the ground substance of connective tissues especially during development when it is known as mucus connective tissue.

   Mucin is soluble in alkaline water and precipitated by acetic acid. We can say that it is a lubricant in animals and in the vegetables. It is connective tissue and its acts as a buffer and a lubricant.

(2) **Mineral Salt:** This is one kind of mineral salt cater neutralizes the acid chime from the stomach.

(3) **Bile Salts:** Bile Salts are chiefly the sodium salts glycochlolic and taurocholic acid. Some potassium salt may also occur to a limited extent. These are soluble in water and Alcohol.

Their solution is distinctly alkaline which control the ph of the Bile juice. They emulsify fats after lowering the surface tension of water they may be regarded such to play important role in the digestive process.

(4) **Bile pigments:** Bile pigments are bilirubin and biliverdin they give distinctive co lour to bile juice. Bilirubin is reddish pigment while biliverdin is greenish Pigment. Bilirubin is converted into biliverdin by mild oxidation while biliverdin is converted into bilirubin by reduction. This pigment can combined with fats because they are having carbonic group in their molecules. They are found probably in form of sodium salt in the bile juice. **Cholesterol:** The Cholesterol in bile juice may be concentrated a product to be excreted the body is an efficient product in it, and is synthesized from acetic acid.

(5) **Lecithin:** It is a typical substance found in the bile juice it is accompanied by trace of soap.

(6) **Fatty & Fatty Acid:** Fatty acids in the carbon changes winches contain no ethylenic or other unsaturated Linkage between carbons, atoms. It is known as not to absorb water or no water soluble.

(7) **Water:** Bile juice contains about 80 to 90 percent of water.

FUNCTION OF BILE JUICE COMBINED

Mostly we know that bile juice is mainly use for digestion of the protein and fats but it has more work.

(1) Maintenance the regulation of body temperature.
(2) Normal water balance of the body.

(3) Maintain the normal reaction of blood in the body.

(4) It's regulating of the normal acid base balance of the duodenum.

(5) It helps the action of all enzymes.

(6) It is important source of. Alkaline for neutralizing the HCL, after entering into the intestine.

(7) It excretes toxin bacteria, heavy metals such as mercury led, bismuth, arsenic, copper, Zink, and drug etc.

1. **Function of mucin or mucus:** It has buffer action its work like antigen and it also works as a lubricant. Mucin helps nerve to work smoothly.

2. **Function of Mineral Salts:** It is of help in digestion and Neutralize the acid enzyme from the Stomach.

3. **Function of Bile salts:** (1) without Function of Bile salt the digestion and absorption of fat is not possible. (2) Bile salt activates pancreatic lipase. (3) Its help in emulsification of food, fats in intestine. In this way bile salt helping the absorption of fats salable vitamin, like A, D, E, K, (4) Bile salts stimulate secretion of more bile from the liver. (5) Bile salt probably in the endogenous synthesis of cholesterol by liver. (6) Bile salt has a mild cathartic (purgative) action (7) Bile salts have an antibacterial action.

4. **Function of Bile pigment:** Bilirubin and biliverdin (1) The bile pigment helps in the formation of hem which is mixed up with the globing part and ultimately forms fresh Hb. (2) A part of the Bile pigment is excreted along with stool as stercibilim While the remaining part gets absorbed and is excreted out by the kidneys as urinary pigments known as urobilline uroerythrinee and urochome. (3) The bile pigments facilitate the absorption of Iron. And other substance, which are necessary for the synthesis of H.B. (4) The chief macrophages are the endothelial cells of the spleen reticulum cells of in the bone marrow, chuffer cells in the liver and reticulum cells in lymph glands oxidized in the

bile passage to Biliverdin. (5) Bile Rubin normally liberated into the blood by the Macrophages is known as heamo bilirubin which gives the indirect reaction. (6) Bilirubin which has passed through the liver cells. It known as, chole– bilirubin which promotes directs reaction.

5. **Function of Cholesterol:** (1) Cholesterol is one of the important constituents in the structure of cells, where its amount is practically constant. (2) Leucocytes and erythrocytes are rich in cholesterol contents, in reds cells it concentration on cell membrane helps to detoxify the hemolytic effects of substance E.G. bacterial Toxin. (3) Transport of fatty acid in the body mainly takes place as cholesterol esters (4) Cholesterol increases the antigen sensitivity (5) During acute infections the cholesterol associates with defense Mechanism of the body. (6) Cholesterol serves as precursor of colic acid and bile salt formation. Vitamin D three formation and ergo sterol. The latter is converted to active vitamin D by ultra violet rays. (7) In the steroids formation when cholesterol is converted into pregnenolone and then progesterone from this are formed adrenal cortex Harmon's androgens and estrogen. (8) Brain tissue has up to 80% cholesterol white matter being richer in it then gray matter. Thus cholesterol is presumed to be involved in electrical impulses Conductions and insulation mechanism.

6. **Function of Lecithin:** It is purify the blood and remove the inorganic matters.

7. **Function of fatty acid:** (1) Fatty acids are to provide fat cells and other tissue by cyclonic corms. (2) They are also synthesized in the fat depots in which they are stored. (3) They circulate bound to albumins and are major source of energy for many organs. (4) Fatty acid maintains the body temperature.

8. **Function of Water:** To make a liquid or able to flow water plays an important role.

HOW CAN WE USE BILE JUICE

(1) We can give orally or by filling in a capsule.

(2) After drying in sun light or inflame we can make a dose.

(3) We can collect bile juice and if it is possible. We can separate the bile pigment, bile salt cholesterol fatty acid, water etc and we can use the thing according to the need of body because they are very valuable things. By the throwing things we can control many chronic diseases Leukemia, Asthma, Eosinophilia, and Phagocytosis, leucopoiesis, Erythropoiesis anemia and many diseases like coronary heart diseases and diabetes, mellitus diseases.

MAINLY WE SEE MAJOR DISEASES

(1) **The coronary heart diseases:** the greatest killer of human being in modern age is coronary hard diseases. Mainly coronary heart diseases caused by cholesterol accumulation in our blood. It can be cured by bile salts or bile juice by orally. (CoOH).

(2) **Diabetes:** All over the world lot of people is suffering from diabetes. Now a day's lot of patients gets insulin resistant and no medicine can control the sugar only diet control the solution. And all the books giving the knowledge the cause of diabetes is unknown and until now diabetes treated by insulin, Tolbutamide, glycozide metformin etc.

Diabetes is known as pancreatic diseases: So it is necessary to know the structure functions and enzymes secreted by pancreas. The pancreas is pale yellow gland which is found in the region of the junction between the stomach and the duodenum. This has certain specialized granular cells that seem to be developed as specialized. Over growths of the gut ermdodrum histological from the rest of the pancreas tissue. The cells are endocrine in function. They have been known as islets cells of Langerhans. These islets cells were not connected to the duct system through which the digestive pancreatic juice flows instead their secretions are freed into the blood circulation. There are three kinds of cells present in islets cells.

(1) Alpha cells or a cell are fairly numerous in most islets their granules are soluble in water, But not in Alcohol.
(2) Beta cells or B cells are smaller and usually more numerous their granules are coarser but alcohol soluble.
(3) Delta cells or D cells are the rarest of the cells present in islet cells.

FUNCTION OF THREE CELLS PRESENT IN THE ISLET CELLS

(1) **Alpha cells:** The cell secrets glucagon's this Harmon converts liver glycogen to glucose.
(2) **Beta cells:** This cells secret insulin the function of insulin to convert excess blood glucose into glycogen that is stored in the liver.
(3) **Delta cells:** The cells produce gas tin it is similar to the Harmon's produce by the stomach it is very small in amount.
   As we know the beta cells of pancreas secret insulin.

Insulin contains three types' enzymes:

(1) **Amylase:** Amylase converts all starches into maltose.
(2) **Trypsin:** Trypsin converts peptones into amino acid
(3) **Lipase:** Lipase converts fat into glycerol and fatty acids. Up till now diabetes treated as:

Definition of diabetes: It is a clinical syndrome. Characterized mainly by polyuria, polydipsia, and polyphagia due to absolute deficiency of insulin or diminished biologic effectiveness of it or both.

Up till now no drug enzymes Harmon's can cure the diabetes only they can control the diabetes. When it is chronic that time all the drugs get resistance. And they are affecting less and now a day the all drugs gets Failure and diabetic patients are in lot of trouble and lot of people die in early stage.

According to my observation knowledge and innovation by useless things bile juice we can solve the many incurable chronic and specific diseases and control and solve some unsolved questions.

All over the world bile juice of animal birds and aquatic creatures thrown useless like anything and all the people are cutting a way the gall bladder of every creature very carefully because they think that it is poison. It is fact that this is bitter in taste and if it is broken down the whole taste becomes bitter. But up till now l does not know why people of the world are not using bile juice, as a natural tonic or as a medicine and why is not preparing the medicine including the bile juice substance because, it is pure and purified by natural process of the body and produce by largest gland (liver) and collect in gall bladder. And its juice work in digestive system.

Every gland secretion depends upon its secretion and bone marrow is also affected by the secretion. It can improve the immunity power of the body because bile has one kind of antigen and it can help to keep the human healthy and it can increase the life of human.

I am sorry to inform you that up till now we have not developed the process to know the bile salt in the blood the normal bile salt in the blood less or excess. We know during Jaundice the bile salt in the blood increases and it can be proved by testing urine or blood. So up till know it is a challenge to world scientist to know the normal value of bile salt in the blood and the combination of COOH + HCl.

MY PREVIOUS DEFINITION OF DIABETES

The deficiency of secret in, bile salt and cyst in (sulpher) in the blood and less of bile juice not secreted by gall bladder or not prepared by liver by Obstruction dehydration fasting malaria typhoid, Kalazar and any other reaction causes diabetes.

Up till now people are using insulin to control the diabetes and other drug also but now a day in lot of patients gets insulin resistance let are failures to simulate the beta cells or pancreas as a whole. The stimulatory and secretary activities of pancreas or Alfa cells beta cells and delta cells depend upon that how much it can get nutrition's. The main nutrition's of pancreas is secretin & bile salts through the blood. When we eat food that time duodenal mucosa secretes a Substance called secretin and same time bile juice is also secreted by the gall bladder both of substance work to digest the food and again they observed by small intestine and mixed with blood and through the blood it conveyed to pancreas and then pancreas secrets glucagons insulin and gastine. This secretion is needed for digesting the food and also' for the whole metabolisms of the body and failure of above mechanism deficiency of insulin takes place and lack of insulin the carbohydrate (glucose) not converted into fat and sugar increase in the blood and strength of the body becomes less and human are getting giddiness and after some times the sugar come in muscles skin eye ear and nerve Nephron cardiac mussels sex Harmon's lymphatic glands will be affected. And the capacity of urinary bladder is lost to control the urine for more time and heal process of body is also disturbed.

According to my thinking when beta cells of pancreas fail to secret insulin that time Alpha cells and delta cells get more strength and they produce More gas tin and Glucagon's. because Diabetic patients have more appetite and also it is in nature that if a person gets loss one hand that time one hand become more strength due to misbalance of secretin. And bile salts Diabetes take place.

If we able to correct it The misbalance we can cure the diabetes by giving good protein diet and after that Bile salts because, when we are eating good protein diet that time, secretin and Bile Salt secret more. If by the liver bile salts are not produce properly. That time we can give by Bile Salts orally then after some time the balance of secretin and Bile Salts become in balance after that not need to take any medicine for diabetes.

Insulin is very use full from the beginning stage it is easily available in every part of market and many kind of herbal combination and medicine but all medicine fail to cure.

MATERIAL METHOD

REFERENCES

1. 1 mL of bile Juice with sugar of milk a single dose for one week.
2. I prepare mother tincture of goat bile juice. 50% of bile juice, 50% Rectified Sprite (ethanol) and kept for 15 days and after that I filtered and kept in bottle. One drop daily for one week or as required.
3. We can use as a injection

Sign Sohail Ahmed (changed Name)
Senior Section Engineer Engg. Dept.(ECR), Sugauli

I, Asha Rani Lal, was suffering with a disease in which my blood does not get clotted from 28 long years. The blood would come out with such tremendensity that it would reach to a height from one and half feet to two feet. I had almost 90 tablets of Vitamin K. but the disease was same as before. At last by having 3 dose of medicine invented in 1998 by Mr. Pramod Stephen I was completely cured. Also the deficiency of blood was also cured. I did not have any tablets of Vitamin K after that and I am also fit till now. The blood clotting has started to form.

Primary School,
Sugali bazaar, East Champaran,

My Publish Articles

The Oxford History of the Laws of England: 1483-1558
Front Cover
John Hamilton Baker
Oxford University Press, 2003 - Law - 964 pages
1 Review

This volume covers the years 1483-1558, a period of immense social, political, and intellectual changes, which profoundly affected the law and its workings. It first considers constitutional developments, and addresses the question of whether there was a rule of law under king Henry VIII. In a period of supposed despotism, and enhanced parliamentary power, protection of liberty was increasing and habeas corpus was emerging. The volume considers the extent to which the law was affected by the intellectual changes of the Renaissance, and how far the English experience differed from that of the Continent. It includes a study of the myriad jurisdictions in Tudor England and their workings; and examines important procedural changes in the central courts, which represent a revolution in the way that cases were presented and decided. The legal profession, its education, its functions, and its literature are examined, and the impact of printing upon legal learning and the role of case-law in comparison with law-school doctrine are addressed. The volume then considers the law itself. Criminal law was becoming more focused during this period as a result of doctrinal exposition in the inns of court and occasional reports of trials. After major conflicts with the Church, major adjustments were made to the benefit of clergy, and the privilege of sanctuary was all but abolished. The volume examines the law of persons in detail, addressing the impact of the abolition of monastic status, the virtual disappearance of village, developments in the law of corporations, and some remarkable statements about the equality of women. The history of private law during this period is dominated by real property and particularly the Statutes of Uses and Wills (designed to protect the king's feudal income against the consequences of trusts) which are given a new interpretation. Leaseholders and copyholders came to be treated as full landowners with rights assimilated to those of freeholders. The land law of the time was highly sophisticated, and becoming more so, but it was only during this period that the beginnings of a law of chattels became discernible. There were also significant changes in the law of contract and tort, not least in the development of a satisfactory remedy for recovering debts.

More »More"

Preview this book"
What people are saying

aged more than 100 years old were awarded with "SatauSamman" in Neelkanth 125 KM from Jamunia Talab Dist. Shihor in Madhya Pradesh India. When they were asked to say about the reason of their long life, they told at different places that honesty, restless, co-operation; routine life and taking food at time are the secret of their long life.

25

OTHER BENEFITS OF CHEWING PROCESS

I READ AND SHOW MANY books on Human & Animal physiology of various writers in National and International editions. They describe their own way. The composition of Saliva there is small difference between books. Now I describe the composition of Saliva according free encyclopedia, the use of Saliva by our forefather and according to me and experience of other people benefited with Saliva.

Saliva is a watery substance located in the mouth of organisms, secreted by the salivary glands. Human saliva is composed of 99% water, while the other 1% consists of electrolytes, mucus, glycoprotein, enzymes, and antibacterial compounds such as secretary IgA and lysozyme.

The enzymes found in saliva are essential in beginning the process of digestion of dietary starches and fats. These enzymes also play a role in breaking down food particles entrapped within dental crevices, protecting teeth from bacterial decay. Furthermore, saliva serves a lubricate function, wetting food and permitting the initiation of swallowing, and protecting the mucosal surfaces of the oral cavity from desiccation.

Various species have special uses for saliva that go beyond predigesting. Some swifts use their gummy saliva to build nests. Aerodramus nests are prized for use in bird's nest soup. Cobras, vipers, and certain other members of the venom clade hunt with venomous saliva injected by fangs. Some arthropods, such as spiders and caterpillars, create thread from salivary glands.

Herbivores like Cow, Buffalos, goat etc. doing ruminant. Fish and caribhores swallowing food directly. Human child at the time of birth till 6 months they digest their food by Saliva. Which contains every kind of essential enzymes and by the Saliva the metabolic process of child become accurate. While cow, buffalo, goat and many herbivores child do ruminants from the birth because sod given them these kind of digestive and metabolic process. If they not to do ruminant then their stomach will be disturbed and they feel illness. This process continues for whole life. Same like against human no do ruminants but till the grown up the teeth the digestive system and metabolic process take place by the saliva after grown up the teeth then the child able to take the solid food from that time we need to chew. But the child wants to eat hurry up and go for playing. Mother father also want to go for duty so they want that his or her son or daughter eat fast. Then the process of eating fast being and goes up to till death. By this reason many kind of syndrome comes and it will create illness.

Now, I describe the new discovery of items in Saliva. Human Saliva is 99.9% water but it contains many. Important substance including electrolytes, mucus, antibacterial compounds and various enzymes produced by our salivary glands.

1. Water
2. **Electrolytes:** 1. Sodium 2. Potassium 3. Calcium 4. Magnesium **5.** Chloride 6. Bicarbonate 7. Phosphate 8. Iodine.
3. **Mucus:** Mucus in Saliva, Mainly consist of mucopolysaccharides and glycoprotine.
4. **Antibacterial Compounds:** 1. Thiocyanate 2. Hydrogen peroxide 3. Secretary glouline A 4. Epidermal growth factor (E&F)

5. **Various enzymes:** There are three major enzymes found in saliva.

    (a) α-amylase–α-Amylase, or ptyalin, secreted by the acinar cells of the parotid and submandibular glands, starts the digestion of starch before the food is even swallowed. It has pH optima of 7.4.

    (b) Lingual lipase. Lingual lipase, which is secreted by the acinar cells of the sublingual gland, has a pH optimum ~4.0 so it is not activated until entering the acidic environment of the stomach.

    (c) Kallikrein. Kallikrein is an enzyme that proteolytically cleaves high-molecular-weight kininogen to produce bradykinin, which is a vasodilator. It is secreted by the acinar cells of all three major salivary glands.

    (d) Antimicrobial enzymes that kill bacteria.

        (i) Lysozyme
        (ii) Salivary lactoperoxidase
        (iii) Lactoferrin
        (iv) Immunoglobulin A

Proline-rich proteins (function in enamel formation, Ca^{2+}-binding, microbe killing and lubrication).

Minor enzymes include salivary acid phosphatases $A + B$, N-acetylmuramoyl-L-alanine amidase, NAD(P)H dehy- drogenase (quinone), superoxide dismutase, glutathione transferase, class 3 aldehyde dehydrogenase, glucose- 6-phosphate isomerase, and tissue kallikrein (function unknown).

Cells: Possibly as much as 8 million human and 500 million bacterial cells per ml. The presence of bacterial products (small organic acids, amines, and thiols) causes saliva to sometimes exhibit foul odor.

Opiorphin, a newly researched pain-killing substance found in human saliva.

BLOOD CLOTTING FACTORS

By these facts we know that in our saliva there are many enzymes and other substance founded. Now I can describe that by chewing we can cure our disease, clinical syndrome and develop our immunity power.

1. As in or saliva nerve growth factor is present, by this way we can develop our sensitiveness and mind power (IQ).
2. Our saliva has anti-bacterial substance. By this way we can put ourselves some bacteria free and we can increase our immunity power.

Now by these facts we know that in our Saliva. Nerve Growth factor is present. If we are able to control and develop our saliva, by doing the masticate process then our nerve & brain will be more active and our IQ power will be increased.

In our Saliva, Proline Protein is present. By this process we can make our teeth strong, beautiful and brighter. This protein is able to produce enamel, which is present in our upper surface of teeth.

Opiorphin is also present in our Saliva. It is a pain killing substance if we will protect our saliva then we can prevent ourselves by any kind of pain like backache, headache, romantic arthritis, gout will be not affecting our body parts.

In our Saliva, blood clotting factor is also presents. Many people are suffering by this problem. If there is a small cut in their body then their blood will not clot. We can cure it by chewing method only.

Gastin is also present in our Saliva; by these enzymes we can develop our test and other hormonal functions. Iodine is also present in our saliva. Iodine & antibacterial compounds can prevent the all types of tumor, abnormal growth of cells, in any part of the body and thyroid problem also.

Epidermal growth factors are also presents in our saliva which is responsible for skins. It is my personal experience that in winter season my body skins get creaked. It is continued till now. In summer season or hot places it disappears. I show myself too many doctors. Doctors' advise me that it is not curable by medicine. There is no treatment in our life. After two or three generations the treatment may come.my self-experiment on my body by new herbs, I bring it and boil it and bathing. I also bring herbs and cooked it in oil and massage in whole body but till now, I not got any relief.

I can say by my own experiment and experience, when I start my chewing process, till that time my skin gets less creaks and there is little brightness on face. Now I can say with full confidence that in our saliva skin or epidermal growth factor is presents. If all people eat water and food by more chewing, then their skin become more shining and they look more beautiful than before. If mother and father will do the above process than coming generation will be healthy, beautiful, attractive and intelligent. Also they will get chewing process by genes. New we know that the function and composition of saliva than we must save or protect our saliva and do not spit here and there and make dirtiness.

The position and composition of saliva changed time to time. Morning, afternoon, evening and night time. When we are in thinking angry, thirsty, hunger, worries and sorrow that time the position of mouth and saliva is also changed and many times we feel dryness of mouth, that time the whole system of our body gets disturbed. When we are happy or in jolly mood then feel very easy in every part of the body. The impact of the season is also effects our body and endocrinal glands. If we put chocolate in our mouth then salivary glands increase their functions but when we drink alcohol, smoke that time the function of salivary glands get disturbed. I heard by my Father, Mother and fore father that if hair of head falls, then people can use the morning saliva and cream of tong will use in bald scaled headed then hair will come up. "Shihuli" (A kind of skin disease) hypo pigment it can cure by saliva. I can tell by my own experiment and other people experiment that by chewing process they get very easy stool, piles cure it, skin becomes healthy and shining, memory power also increase. They feel painless and by this way we know that by chewing process there are too many kind of benefits.

Eat food and water by chewing more
make yourself and your generation disease free.

26

············ ✑ ············

DISCUSSION

Make your teeth & skin pretty, Make your brain straight full.
Nobody wants to die
Death is must
live with joyful life
age become years
to years who live healthy in life,
He is happiest person.

I HAVE GIVEN MY BOOK to many people. Many people get benefits that follow my methods but there are who do not believe on this method because they are done using it in a few days and left the process because they want quick result. Lipase completely different from pancreatic amylase & lipase then I asked that from the birth of a child till 6 months the function of pancreases of a child not working at all. How the carbohydrates and fat metabolism take place that mean God gave us an accurate alternative system for our metabolism.

I want to tell readers that during 6 month the metabolic process of all enzymes secreted by pancreases fulfill by salivary enzymes.

By above matters we must know that in our body, God gave us different method to keep our metabolism fit and accurate but we do not know that method so we become sick and troubled. So, I request all you must follow books method continue for 3 months then you will find good result.

27

THE IMPACT OF MEDICINE

NOW WE WILL SEE THE impact of many medical pathy will work in our body and Metabolic process.

Food—Food is very necessary for our body. Everybody knows that without food then we cannot image of life. When we take Balance diet we get necessary vitamin and mineral salt and other substance necessary for our body If one substance is less then, It will complete by other source for some time but if it is continues for long time then deficiency of substance come out by the same cause and for next the process of metabolic disturbance occur in our body and we feel severe disease or disturbance. Flower's fruity vegetable, grain, pulse, egg, meat, fish, stem cane root leaf each and every part have other substance and different plant have different substance in different quantity. For this reason we must take all kind of above describe food substance. Today we see that only we are cultivating or eating which is more yielding. More in weight and which is easily available in market and we are using new method and utensils, old system utensils system food systems and living standard completely changed as—Marua, Kodo, china, sweet potato, Bulbous root (Diossoria) suthani, is now out of our cultivated area and it is not available in any market fasciculate. After very few times looking in market by this reason the substance present in these things our body will not get. I heard by old people that we must eat these things once in a year by eating these things the any kind of tumor will not develop in the body by this reason many kind of disease develop in our body and now a day the problem is just like epidemic.

Exercise & Yoga–Exercise and yoga is very necessary to keep our body healthy, we know that there are many kind of yoga which impact and activate our different organs. But it cannot provide the deficiency of our body and not able to give strength by yoga and exercise we can keep our body active. By this process we can burn our energy. If we take an example of diabetes patients, then we found that by exercise & yoga by burning energy we can control sugar but cannot fill the insulin and other substance. When we want to keep ours elf healthy then we must exercise along with balance diet with more chew by this way if any vitamin or mineral salt lacking in food which is fulfill by our saliva.

Medicine & Substitute–When we fall ill we must need medicine to increase our immunity power and sometime decrease it. Some medicine are very useful to kill bacteria, Bacillus etc. but when our immunity power become less then the passions of our body is very dangerous. We know that we have immunity power to fight against many germs which can keep us healthy without medicine today we see that if a person get diabetes or thyroid problem and his or her pancreas and thyroid gland do not work properly then medical world advise him or her to take Insulin and thyroid pills whole life by this way our body become depend on that substance sometime this substance increase and decrease in our body and our metabolic process disturb by this process and we feel trouble.

Other treatment system and other instruments–Today in our world there are many medical and non-medical path and different kind of instrument. New research is going on which is stem cell process and cells division changes process are examples.

Medicine analysis change of combinations is continued from the old age. But I want to say with full confidence that It cannot fill the deficiency of our body or not correct our metabolism, because we see that If we increase one side then next side will be less our body needs different medicine for different human we cannot apply one medicine for all human and we are not able to say that, this man need this much medicine. We know that what the substance is found and needed for leaving creature and how to fulfill it but how much he or she needed this medicine we cannot know the exact amount. We ask patients and stop the medicine. If accurate we will take an example of obesity then we can find that obesity is due to more reason. For example, eating more food its gets metabolic disorder' hypothalamus, hyper thyroid and hypothyroid deficiency. Iron deficiency diabetic condition, but when we study we find that some people that I eat very less even then I am vary fatty and Against that very thin people eat very much but they are not fatty. Fatty people eat very less but his body becomes more weighted. When we see mother & father they give more food to their children in I see by my own eyes that many mothers beat their children for eating mother and father think that If her children eat more than her children will be healthy, but against it her children became fatty and the habit of more eating and the child become more fatty and due to heavy weight child not able to walk freely and not able to play, by this reason some time child get severe illness and he feels mental weakness and due to heavy weight and fat the metabolic process are also changed. If this process continue for long time then this habit transfer by gens to next generations now. It is an epidemic in the word so my advice to all people to give limited food to the children as they require don't force them for eating more food. Must be full of vitamins and minerals as a balance diet and teach them for more chew process by childhood, food & water also by this process they will be free from many disease, they get more immunity power and they will be healthy. Handsome and wise all things they will get by nature.

My next books are:

1. The power of our mouth
2. ----------

www.ingramcontent.com/pod-product-compliance
Lightning Source LLC
Chambersburg PA
CBHW060109300526
45791CB00018B/870